VEGETARIAN SJOGREN SYNDROME COOKBOOK FOR BEGINNERS

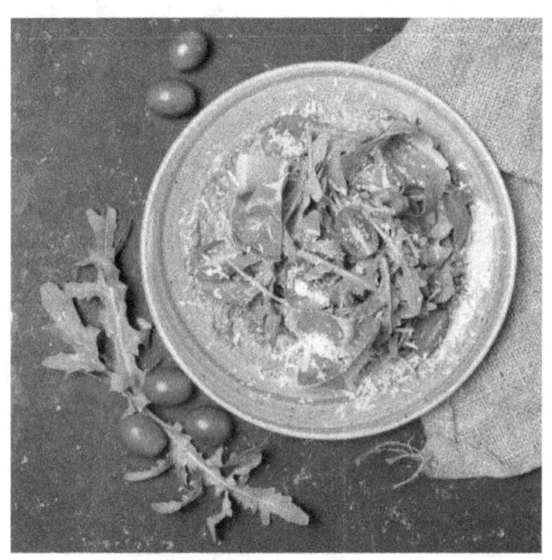

DR. JESSICA SMITH

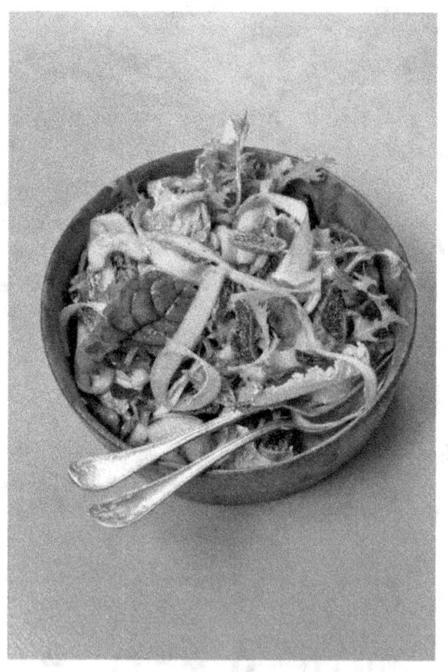

TABLE OF CONTENTS

CHAPTER ONE

How to Use this Cookbook

Understanding Sjogren's Syndrome:

Familiarize yourself with the basics of Sjogren's syndrome, including common symptoms such as dry mouth, dry eyes, and fatigue, to better understand how diet can play a role in managing these symptoms.

Explore Vegetarian Ingredients:

Begin by exploring a variety of vegetarian ingredients such as fruits, vegetables, whole grains, legumes, nuts, seeds, and plant-based proteins like tofu and tempeh, which form the foundation of a Sjogren-friendly diet.

Stock Up on Essentials:

Ensure your pantry is stocked with essential ingredients such as olive oil, herbs, spices, and low-sodium vegetable broth to add flavor to your dishes without relying on excessive salt.

Start with Simple Recipes: Begin your culinary journey with simple and beginner-friendly recipes that require minimal ingredients and preparation time, such as salads, soups, and stir-fries.

Hydration is Key:

Focus on incorporating hydrating foods like water-rich fruits (watermelon, oranges), vegetables (cucumber, celery), and soups to combat dry mouth and eyes, common symptoms of Sjogren's syndrome.

Experiment with Flavors:

Experiment with a variety of herbs, spices, and condiments to add depth and complexity to your dishes, enhancing their flavor without compromising on health.

Balance Your Plate:

Aim to create balanced meals that include a mix of carbohydrates, protein, healthy fats, and plenty of colorful fruits and vegetables to ensure you're getting a wide range of nutrients.

Meal Planning and Preparation: Take time to plan your meals and prepare ingredients in advance to streamline the cooking process and make healthier choices throughout the week.

Listen to Your Body:

Pay attention to how different foods make you feel and adjust your diet accordingly. Keep a food diary to track any triggers or patterns that may exacerbate symptoms.

Seek Support and Guidance:

Don't hesitate to seek support and guidance from healthcare professionals, including registered dietitians, who can provide personalized recommendations and support on your journey to better health with Sjogren's syndrome.

Understanding Vegetarian Sjogren Syndrome for Beginners

Understanding vegetarian Sjogren's syndrome for beginners is the first step towards effectively managing this autoimmune condition through diet.

Sjogren's syndrome primarily affects the moisture-producing glands, leading to symptoms such as dry mouth, dry eyes, and fatigue.

A vegetarian approach to managing this condition focuses on consuming plant-based foods rich in nutrients that support overall health and alleviate symptoms.

Beginners should familiarize themselves with the principles of a vegetarian diet, emphasizing fruits, vegetables, whole grains, legumes, nuts, seeds, and plant-based proteins.

These foods provide essential vitamins, minerals, antioxidants, and fiber, which are beneficial for immune function and reducing inflammation associated with Sjogren's syndrome.

Hydration is a critical aspect of managing Sjogren's syndrome, and beginners should focus on incorporating hydrating foods like water-rich fruits and vegetables, soups, and herbal teas into their diet to combat dryness symptoms effectively.

Furthermore, beginners should experiment with flavors, herbs, and spices to enhance the taste of their meals without relying on excessive salt.

Balancing meals with a variety of nutrients and listening to the body's cues are also essential aspects of understanding and adapting to a vegetarian Sjogren's syndrome diet.

Seeking guidance from healthcare professionals, including registered dietitians, can provide beginners with personalized recommendations and support as they navigate their journey towards better health with Sjogren's syndrome.

Principles of Vegetarian Sjogren Syndrome for Beginners

For beginners navigating a vegetarian diet tailored to Sjogren's syndrome, understanding the fundamental principles is crucial for effectively managing symptoms and promoting overall well-being.

Here are the key principles to guide beginners:

Hydration Focus: Prioritize hydration by incorporating water-rich fruits and vegetables, herbal teas, and hydrating soups into meals. Hydration is essential for combating dry mouth and eyes, common symptoms of Sjogren's syndrome.

Nutrient-Rich Foods: Emphasize whole, plant-based foods such as fruits, vegetables, whole grains, legumes, nuts, and seeds.

These foods provide essential vitamins, minerals, antioxidants, and fiber necessary for supporting immune function and reducing inflammation associated with Sjogren's syndrome.

Omega-3 Fatty Acids: Include sources of omega-3 fatty acids such as flaxseeds, chia seeds, walnuts, and algae-based supplements to help reduce inflammation and alleviate symptoms.

Protein Sources: Incorporate plant-based protein sources like tofu, tempeh, lentils, and beans to support muscle health and overall nutrition without relying on animal products.

Oral Health Support: Choose crunchy fruits and vegetables like apples, carrots, and celery to stimulate saliva production and maintain oral hygiene, reducing the risk of dental issues associated with Sjogren's syndrome.

Minimize Inflammatory Foods: Limit intake of processed foods, refined sugars, and saturated fats, as they can exacerbate inflammation and worsen symptoms. Focus on whole, unprocessed plant-based foods instead.

Consultation with Healthcare Professionals: Seek guidance from healthcare professionals, including registered dietitians, to tailor the diet plan to individual needs and ensure it complements treatment and supports overall health effectively.

Benefits of Vegetarian Sjogren Syndrome for Beginners

Embracing a vegetarian diet tailored to beginners with Sjogren's syndrome offers a multitude of benefits that can positively impact their overall health and well-being.

Here are some key advantages:

Reduced Inflammation: A plant-based diet is naturally anti-inflammatory, rich in antioxidants, vitamins, and minerals found in fruits, vegetables, whole grains, and legumes.

This can help mitigate inflammation associated with Sjogren's syndrome, alleviating symptoms such as joint pain and fatigue.

Improved Hydration: Vegetarian diets typically include hydrating foods like water-rich fruits and vegetables, soups, and herbal teas, which can effectively combat dry mouth and dry eyes, common symptoms of Sjogren's syndrome.

Nutrient Density: Plant-based foods are packed with essential nutrients, including vitamins, minerals, fiber, and antioxidants, which are crucial for supporting immune function, reducing oxidative stress, and promoting overall health.

Heart Health: By focusing on plant-based sources of protein and healthy fats, such as nuts, seeds, and legumes, beginners can support heart health and reduce the risk of cardiovascular disease associated with Sjogren's syndrome.

Weight Management: Vegetarian diets tend to be lower in calories and saturated fats while being higher in fiber, which can aid in weight management and reduce the risk of obesity-related conditions.

Oral Health Support: Crunchy fruits and vegetables included in a vegetarian diet can stimulate saliva production, promoting oral hygiene and reducing the risk of dental issues associated with Sjogren's syndrome.

Enhanced Digestion: Plant-based diets are rich in fiber, which supports digestive health, regulates bowel movements, and alleviates symptoms such as constipation commonly experienced by individuals with Sjogren's syndrome.

By embracing the benefits of a vegetarian diet tailored to beginners with Sjogren's syndrome, individuals can experience improvements in symptom management, overall health, and quality of life.

It's essential to consult with healthcare professionals to ensure the diet plan meets individual nutritional needs and complements treatment strategies effectively.

Tips for Vegetarian Sjogren Syndrome for Beginners

For beginners embarking on a vegetarian diet tailored to manage Sjogren's syndrome, it's essential to approach the transition with practical tips and strategies to ensure success and symptom management. Here are some helpful tips:

Educate Yourself: Learn about Sjogren's syndrome and how dietary choices can impact symptoms. Understanding the condition and its dietary implications is crucial for making informed choices.

Gradual Transition: Transitioning to a vegetarian diet gradually can make the adjustment smoother. Start by incorporating more plant-based meals into your diet while gradually reducing animal products.

Hydration Focus: Prioritize hydration by consuming plenty of water-rich fruits and vegetables, herbal teas, and hydrating soups to combat dry mouth and eyes, common symptoms of Sjogren's syndrome.

Explore Variety: Experiment with a wide range of vegetarian ingredients, recipes, and cuisines to keep meals interesting and flavorful. Embrace new foods and cooking techniques to discover what works best for you.

Plan Ahead: Take time to plan your meals and snacks in advance to ensure you have nutritious options readily available. Meal prepping can help save time and make healthier choices throughout the week.

Focus on Whole Foods: Emphasize whole, unprocessed plant-based foods such as fruits, vegetables, whole grains, legumes, nuts, and seeds. These foods provide essential nutrients and support overall health.

Seek Support: Join online communities, forums, or support groups for individuals with Sjogren's syndrome or those following a vegetarian diet.

Connecting with others can provide valuable tips, encouragement, and support on your journey.

Listen to Your Body: Pay attention to how different foods make you feel and adjust your diet accordingly. Keep a food diary to track any triggers or patterns that may exacerbate symptoms.

Consult with Healthcare Professionals: Seek guidance from healthcare professionals, including registered dietitians, who can provide personalized recommendations and support tailored to your individual needs and health goals.

Be Patient and Flexible: Remember that transitioning to a new diet takes time and patience. Be kind to yourself and allow for flexibility as you navigate this journey. Focus on progress rather than perfection, and celebrate small victories along the way.

Guidelines for Vegetarian Sjogren Syndrome for Beginners

For beginners exploring a vegetarian diet tailored to managing Sjogren's syndrome, following guidelines can provide structure and support in making informed dietary choices.

Here are essential guidelines to consider:

Educate Yourself: Learn about Sjogren's syndrome and how dietary choices can impact symptoms. Understanding the condition and its dietary implications is crucial for making informed decisions.

Hydration Priority: Prioritize hydration by consuming hydrating foods like water-rich fruits and vegetables, herbal teas, and soups. Staying adequately hydrated helps alleviate dry mouth and eyes, common symptoms of Sjogren's syndrome.

Nutrient-Rich Foods: Emphasize whole, plant-based foods such as fruits, vegetables, whole grains, legumes, nuts, and seeds. These foods are rich in essential vitamins, minerals, antioxidants, and fiber, supporting overall health and symptom management.

Omega-3 Fatty Acids: Include sources of omega-3 fatty acids like flaxseeds, chia seeds, walnuts, and algae-based supplements to help reduce inflammation and alleviate symptoms associated with Sjogren's syndrome.

Balanced Meals: Aim for balanced meals that include a variety of nutrients, including carbohydrates, protein, healthy fats, vitamins, and minerals. Focus on incorporating colorful fruits and vegetables into each meal.

Limit Inflammatory Foods: Minimize intake of processed foods, refined sugars, and saturated fats, as they can exacerbate inflammation and worsen symptoms. Opt for whole, unprocessed plant-based foods instead.

Meal Planning: Take time to plan your meals and snacks in advance to ensure you have nutritious options readily available. Meal prepping can help save time and make healthier choices throughout the week.

Consult with Healthcare Professionals: Seek guidance from healthcare professionals, including registered dietitians, who can provide personalized recommendations and support tailored to your individual needs and health goals.

Listen to Your Body: Pay attention to how different foods make you feel and adjust your diet accordingly. Keep a food diary to track any triggers or patterns that may exacerbate symptoms.

Be Patient and Flexible: Remember that transitioning to a new diet takes time and patience.

Be kind to yourself and allow for flexibility as you navigate this journey. Focus on progress rather than perfection, and celebrate small victories along the way.

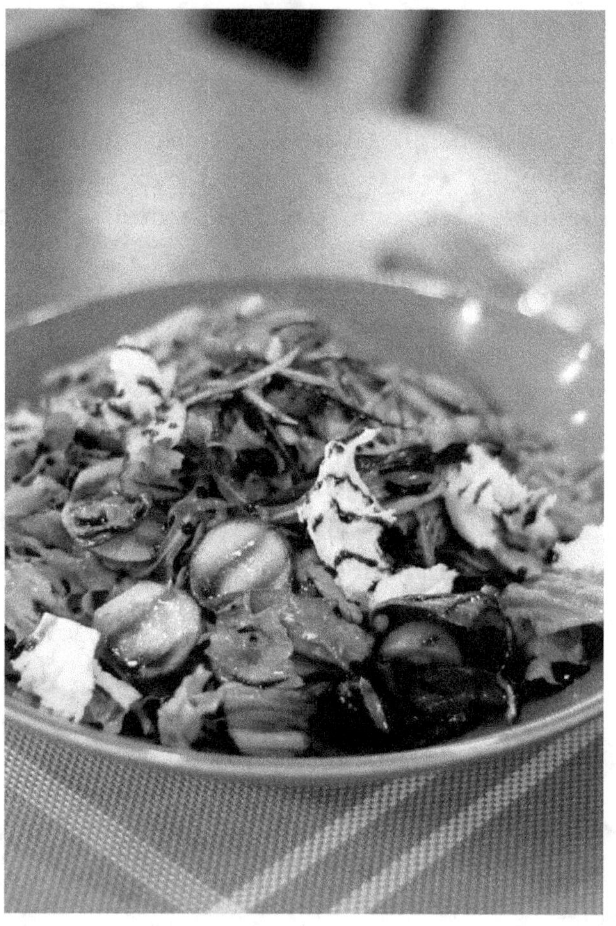

CHAPTER TWO

1: Berry Spinach Smoothie

Ingredients:

- ➢ 1 cup spinach leaves
- ➢ 1/2 cup mixed berries (strawberries, blueberries, raspberries)
- ➢ 1/2 banana
- ➢ 1/2 cup plain Greek yogurt (or plant-based yogurt for vegan option)
- ➢ 1/2 cup water or almond milk
- ➢ 1 tablespoon chia seeds (optional)

Instructions:

- ➢ Place all ingredients in a blender.
- ➢ Blend until smooth.
- ➢ Serve immediately.

Health Benefits: This smoothie is rich in antioxidants, vitamins, and minerals from spinach and berries, supporting immune function and hydration. Greek yogurt provides probiotics for gut health.

Preparation Time: 5 minutes

2: Avocado and Tomato Toast

Ingredients:

- ➢ 1 ripe avocado
- ➢ 2 slices whole grain bread
- ➢ 1 small tomato, sliced
- ➢ Salt and pepper to taste
- ➢ Optional: red pepper flakes or fresh basil for garnish

Instructions:

- ➢ Toast the bread slices until golden brown.
- ➢ Mash the avocado and spread it evenly on the toast.
- ➢ Top with sliced tomato.
- ➢ Season with salt, pepper, and any desired garnishes.
- ➢ Serve immediately.

Health Benefits:

- ➢ Avocado provides healthy fats, while tomatoes offer vitamins and antioxidants.
- ➢ Whole grain bread adds fiber for digestion.

Preparation Time: 10 minutes

3: Quinoa Salad

Ingredients:

- ➢ 1 cup cooked quinoa
- ➢ 1/2 cup chickpeas, rinsed and drained
- ➢ 1/2 cucumber, diced
- ➢ 1/2 bell pepper, diced
- ➢ 1/4 cup diced red onion
- ➢ 1/4 cup chopped fresh parsley
- ➢ Juice of 1 lemon
- ➢ 2 tablespoons olive oil
- ➢ Salt and pepper to taste

Instructions:

- ➢ In a large bowl, combine cooked quinoa, chickpeas, cucumber, bell pepper, red onion, and parsley.
- ➢ Drizzle with lemon juice and olive oil.
- ➢ Season with salt and pepper.
- ➢ Toss until well combined.
- ➢ Serve chilled or at room temperature.

Health Benefits:

> Quinoa provides protein and fiber, while vegetables offer vitamins and antioxidants.
> Olive oil adds healthy fats for heart health.

Preparation Time: 15 minutes

4: Lentil Soup

Ingredients:

> 1 cup dried green lentils, rinsed
> 1 onion, diced
> 2 carrots, diced
> 2 celery stalks, diced
> 2 cloves garlic, minced
> 6 cups vegetable broth
> 1 teaspoon dried thyme
> 1 teaspoon dried rosemary
> Salt and pepper to taste
> Fresh parsley for garnish

Instructions:

> In a large pot, sauté onion, carrots, celery, and garlic until softened.

- ➢ Add lentils, vegetable broth, thyme, and rosemary.
- ➢ Bring to a boil, then reduce heat and simmer for 20-25 minutes until lentils are tender.
- ➢ Season with salt and pepper.
- ➢ Serve hot, garnished with fresh parsley.

Health Benefits:

- ➢ Lentils are rich in protein and fiber, supporting digestive health and providing sustained energy.
- ➢ Vegetables add vitamins and minerals.

Preparation Time: 30 minutes

5: Chickpea Stir-Fry

Ingredients:

- ➢ 1 can chickpeas, drained and rinsed
- ➢ 2 cups mixed vegetables (bell peppers, broccoli, snap peas)
- ➢ 2 cloves garlic, minced
- ➢ 2 tablespoons soy sauce (or tamari for gluten-free option)
- ➢ 1 tablespoon sesame oil
- ➢ Cooked brown rice for serving

Instructions:

> Heat sesame oil in a large skillet over medium heat.
> Add garlic and sauté until fragrant.
> Add mixed vegetables and chickpeas. Cook until vegetables are tender-crisp.
> Stir in soy sauce and cook for another minute.
> Serve over cooked brown rice.

Health Benefits:

> Chickpeas provide protein and fiber, while vegetables offer vitamins and antioxidants.
> Brown rice adds complex carbohydrates for sustained energy.

Preparation Time: 20 minutes

6: Sweet Potato and Black Bean Tacos

Ingredients:

> 2 medium sweet potatoes, peeled and diced
> 1 can black beans, rinsed and drained
> 1 teaspoon chili powder
> 1/2 teaspoon cumin
> Salt and pepper to taste

- ➢ 8 small corn tortillas
- ➢ Toppings: diced avocado, salsa, shredded lettuce, lime wedges

Instructions:

- ➢ Preheat oven to 400°F (200°C).
- ➢ Toss sweet potatoes with chili powder, cumin, salt, and pepper.
- ➢ Spread sweet potatoes on a baking sheet and roast for 20-25 minutes until tender.
- ➢ In a separate skillet, heat black beans until warmed through.
- ➢ Warm tortillas in the oven or on a skillet.
- ➢ Assemble tacos with sweet potatoes, black beans, and desired toppings.
- ➢ Serve with lime wedges.

Health Benefits:

- ➢ Sweet potatoes are rich in vitamins and fiber, while black beans provide protein and minerals.
- ➢ Corn tortillas are gluten-free and high in fiber.

Preparation Time: 30 minutes

Ingredients:

- 8 ounces whole wheat spaghetti
- 2 cups baby spinach
- 1 cup sliced mushrooms
- 2 cloves garlic, minced
- 2 tablespoons olive oil
- Juice of 1 lemon
- Salt and pepper to taste
- Grated Parmesan cheese or nutritional yeast (optional)

Instructions:

- Cook spaghetti according to package instructions.
- In a large skillet, heat olive oil over medium heat.
- Add garlic and mushrooms. Sauté until mushrooms are tender.
- Add spinach and cook until wilted.
- Drain cooked spaghetti and add it to the skillet.
- Drizzle with lemon juice and toss until well combined.
- Season with salt and pepper.

- Serve hot, topped with grated Parmesan cheese or nutritional yeast if desired.

Health Benefits:

- Spinach is high in iron and vitamins, while mushrooms provide antioxidants and fiber.
- Whole wheat pasta adds complex carbohydrates for sustained energy.

Preparation Time: 20 minutes

8: Tofu Vegetable Stir-Fry

Ingredients:

- 1 block firm tofu, pressed and cubed
- 2 cups mixed vegetables (bell peppers, broccoli, snow peas)
- 2 cloves garlic, minced
- 2 tablespoons soy sauce (or tamari for gluten-free option)
- 1 tablespoon sesame oil
- Cooked brown rice for serving

Instructions:

- Heat sesame oil in a large skillet over medium heat.

- ➢ Add tofu cubes and cook until golden brown on all sides.
- ➢ Add garlic and sauté until fragrant.
- ➢ Add mixed vegetables and cook until tender-crisp.
- ➢ Stir in soy sauce and cook for another minute.
- ➢ Serve over cooked brown rice.

Health Benefits:

- ➢ Tofu is a source of plant-based protein, while vegetables provide vitamins and minerals.
- ➢ Brown rice adds fiber and complex carbohydrates.

Preparation Time: 30 minutes

9: Mediterranean Chickpea Salad

Ingredients:

- ➢ 1 can chickpeas, drained and rinsed
- ➢ 1 cucumber, diced
- ➢ 1 tomato, diced
- ➢ 1/4 cup diced red onion
- ➢ 1/4 cup chopped fresh parsley
- ➢ Juice of 1 lemon
- ➢ 2 tablespoons olive oil

➢ Salt and pepper to taste

➢ Optional: crumbled feta cheese or olives for garnish

Instructions:

➢ In a large bowl, combine chickpeas, cucumber, tomato, red onion, and parsley.

➢ Drizzle with lemon juice and olive oil.

➢ Season with salt and pepper.

➢ Toss until well combined.

➢ Garnish with crumbled feta cheese or olives if desired.

➢ Serve chilled or at room temperature.

Health Benefits:

➢ Chickpeas provide protein and fiber, while vegetables offer vitamins and antioxidants.

➢ Olive oil adds healthy fats for heart health.

Preparation Time: 15 minutes

10: Vegetable Curry

Ingredients:

➢ 1 tablespoon coconut oil

➢ 1 onion, diced

- ➢ 2 cloves garlic, minced
- ➢ 2 teaspoons curry powder
- ➢ 1 teaspoon ground turmeric
- ➢ 1 teaspoon ground cumin
- ➢ 1 can coconut milk
- ➢ 2 cups mixed vegetables (carrots, potatoes, cauliflower, peas)
- ➢ Salt and pepper to taste
- ➢ Cooked brown rice for serving

Instructions:

- ➢ Heat coconut oil in a large pot over medium heat.
- ➢ Add onion and garlic. Sauté until softened.
- ➢ Stir in curry powder, turmeric, and cumin. Cook for another minute.
- ➢ Add coconut milk and mixed vegetables. Bring to a simmer.
- ➢ Cover and cook for 15-20 minutes until vegetables are tender.
- ➢ Season with salt and pepper.
- ➢ Serve hot over cooked brown rice.

Health Benefits:

- ➢ Coconut milk adds creaminess and healthy fats, while vegetables provide vitamins, minerals, and fiber.
- ➢ Brown rice adds fiber and complex carbohydrates.

Preparation Time: 30 minutes

11: Lentil Spinach Soup

Ingredients:

- ➢ 1 cup green lentils, rinsed
- ➢ 1 onion, diced
- ➢ 2 carrots, diced
- ➢ 2 celery stalks, diced
- ➢ 2 cloves garlic, minced
- ➢ 6 cups vegetable broth
- ➢ 2 cups fresh spinach leaves
- ➢ 1 teaspoon dried thyme
- ➢ 1 teaspoon dried oregano
- ➢ Salt and pepper to taste
- ➢ Fresh lemon juice for serving

Instructions:

> In a large pot, sauté onion, carrots, celery, and garlic until softened.
> Add lentils, vegetable broth, thyme, and oregano.
> Bring to a boil, then reduce heat and simmer for 20-25 minutes until lentils are tender.
> Add fresh spinach leaves and cook until wilted.
> Season with salt and pepper.
> Serve hot with a squeeze of fresh lemon juice.

Health Benefits:

> Lentils provide protein and fiber, while spinach offers vitamins and antioxidants.
> This soup is hydrating and comforting, perfect for soothing dry mouth and eyes.

Preparation Time: 40 minutes

12: Vegetable Stir-Fried Quinoa

Ingredients:

> 1 cup quinoa, rinsed
> 2 cups water or vegetable broth
> 2 tablespoons olive oil

- 1 onion, diced
- 2 cloves garlic, minced
- 2 cups mixed vegetables (bell peppers, broccoli, carrots)
- 2 tablespoons soy sauce (or tamari for gluten-free option)
- Salt and pepper to taste
- Fresh cilantro for garnish (optional)

Instructions:

- In a saucepan, bring water or vegetable broth to a boil.
- Add quinoa, reduce heat to low, and simmer for 15-20 minutes until quinoa is cooked and liquid is absorbed.
- Heat olive oil in a large skillet over medium heat.
- Add onion and garlic, sauté until fragrant.
- Add mixed vegetables and cook until tender.
- Stir in cooked quinoa and soy sauce. Cook for another 2-3 minutes.
- Season with salt and pepper.
- Garnish with fresh cilantro if desired.
- Serve hot.

Health Benefits:

- ➢ Quinoa is a complete protein and high in fiber, while vegetables provide vitamins and minerals.
- ➢ This dish is nutritious and satisfying, supporting overall health.

Preparation Time: 30 minutes

13: Mediterranean Chickpea Buddha Bowl

Ingredients:

- ➢ 1 cup cooked quinoa or brown rice
- ➢ 1 can chickpeas, drained and rinsed
- ➢ 1 tablespoon olive oil
- ➢ 1 teaspoon smoked paprika
- ➢ 1 teaspoon ground cumin
- ➢ Salt and pepper to taste
- ➢ 2 cups mixed greens (spinach, kale, arugula)
- ➢ 1/2 cucumber, sliced
- ➢ 1/2 cup cherry tomatoes, halved
- ➢ 1/4 cup Kalamata olives, sliced
- ➢ Hummus for serving

Instructions:

> Preheat oven to 400°F (200°C).

> Toss chickpeas with olive oil, smoked paprika, cumin, salt, and pepper.

> Spread chickpeas on a baking sheet and roast for 20-25 minutes until crispy.

> Assemble Buddha bowls with cooked quinoa or brown rice, mixed greens, cucumber, cherry tomatoes, and Kalamata olives.

> Top with roasted chickpeas and a dollop of hummus.

> Serve immediately.

Health Benefits:

> This Buddha bowl is packed with protein, fiber, vitamins, and minerals from chickpeas, quinoa, vegetables, and olives.

> It's a satisfying and nourishing meal option.

Preparation Time: 30 minutes

14: Cauliflower Rice Stir-Fry

Ingredients:

> 1 head cauliflower, grated into rice-like texture

- ➢ 2 tablespoons sesame oil
- ➢ 2 cloves garlic, minced
- ➢ 2 cups mixed vegetables (bell peppers, snap peas, carrots)
- ➢ 2 tablespoons soy sauce (or tamari for gluten-free option)
- ➢ 1 tablespoon rice vinegar
- ➢ 1 tablespoon maple syrup
- ➢ Salt and pepper to taste
- ➢ Sesame seeds for garnish

Instructions:

- ➢ Heat sesame oil in a large skillet over medium heat.
- ➢ Add garlic and sauté until fragrant.
- ➢ Add mixed vegetables and cook until tender-crisp.
- ➢ Stir in cauliflower rice and cook for another 3-4 minutes until heated through.
- ➢ In a small bowl, whisk together soy sauce, rice vinegar, and maple syrup. Pour over the cauliflower rice mixture.
- ➢ Cook for another 2-3 minutes until sauce is absorbed.
- ➢ Season with salt and pepper.
- ➢ Garnish with sesame seeds before serving.

Health Benefits:

> ➤ Cauliflower rice is low in calories and carbohydrates, while vegetables provide vitamins and minerals.
> ➤ This dish is light, flavorful, and suitable for those watching their carbohydrate intake.

Preparation Time: 20 minutes

15: Spinach and Mushroom Quiche

Ingredients:

> ➤ 1 prepared pie crust (store-bought or homemade)
> ➤ 1 tablespoon olive oil
> ➤ 1 onion, diced
> ➤ 2 cups fresh spinach leaves
> ➤ 1 cup sliced mushrooms
> ➤ 6 large eggs
> ➤ 1/2 cup milk (dairy or plant-based)
> ➤ 1/2 cup shredded cheese (cheddar, mozzarella, or dairy-free cheese)
> ➤ Salt and pepper to taste
> ➤ Fresh parsley for garnish

Instructions:

- Preheat oven to 375°F (190°C).
- Heat olive oil in a skillet over medium heat.
- Add onion and sauté until softened.
- Add spinach and mushrooms, cook until wilted and tender.
- In a mixing bowl, whisk together eggs and milk. Season with salt and pepper.
- Place the prepared pie crust in a pie dish. Spread the spinach and mushroom mixture evenly over the crust.
- Pour the egg mixture over the vegetables.
- Sprinkle shredded cheese on top.
- Bake in the preheated oven for 35-40 minutes until the center is set and the crust is golden brown.
- Garnish with fresh parsley before serving.

Health Benefits:

- Spinach is rich in iron and vitamins, while mushrooms provide antioxidants.
- This quiche is protein-packed and makes a satisfying meal option for any time of day.

Preparation Time: 1 hour

16: Chickpea Salad Sandwich

Ingredients:

- ➤ 1 can chickpeas, drained and rinsed
- ➤ 1/4 cup vegan mayonnaise (or regular mayonnaise)
- ➤ 2 tablespoons Dijon mustard
- ➤ 2 tablespoons lemon juice
- ➤ 1/4 cup diced celery
- ➤ 1/4 cup diced red onion
- ➤ 2 tablespoons chopped fresh dill (or 1 teaspoon dried dill)
- ➤ Salt and pepper to taste
- ➤ Whole grain bread or lettuce leaves for serving

Instructions:

- ➤ In a mixing bowl, mash chickpeas with a fork or potato masher until chunky.
- ➤ Add vegan mayonnaise, Dijon mustard, lemon juice, celery, red onion, and dill. Stir until well combined.
- ➤ Season with salt and pepper to taste.
- ➤ Serve chickpea salad on whole grain bread slices or lettuce leaves to make wraps.

> Enjoy immediately or refrigerate for later.

Health Benefits:

> Chickpeas provide protein and fiber, while vegetables offer vitamins and minerals.
> This salad is a nutritious and satisfying alternative to traditional tuna or egg salad sandwiches.

Preparation Time: 15 minutes

17: Stuffed Bell Peppers

Ingredients:

> 4 large bell peppers, halved and seeds removed
> 1 cup cooked quinoa
> 1 can black beans, drained and rinsed
> 1 cup corn kernels (fresh, frozen, or canned)
> 1 cup diced tomatoes
> 1/2 cup diced red onion
> 1 teaspoon chili powder
> 1/2 teaspoon cumin
> Salt and pepper to taste
> Shredded cheese or nutritional yeast for topping

Instructions:

- ➢ Preheat oven to 375°F (190°C).
- ➢ In a large mixing bowl, combine cooked quinoa, black beans, corn, diced tomatoes, red onion, chili powder, cumin, salt, and pepper.
- ➢ Place bell pepper halves in a baking dish, cut side up.
- ➢ Spoon quinoa mixture into each pepper half until filled.
- ➢ Cover the baking dish with aluminum foil and bake for 30-35 minutes until peppers are tender.
- ➢ Remove foil, sprinkle shredded cheese or nutritional yeast on top of each stuffed pepper, and return to the oven for another 5 minutes until cheese is melted.
- ➢ Serve hot.

Health Benefits:

- ➢ Bell peppers are rich in vitamins and antioxidants, while quinoa and black beans provide protein and fiber.
- ➢ This dish is colorful, flavorful, and nutrient-packed.

Preparation Time: 45 minutes

18: Zucchini Noodles with Pesto

Ingredients:

- ➤ 4 medium zucchinis, spiralized into noodles
- ➤ 1 cup fresh basil leaves
- ➤ 1/4 cup pine nuts
- ➤ 2 cloves garlic
- ➤ 1/4 cup grated Parmesan cheese (or nutritional yeast for vegan option)
- ➤ 1/4 cup olive oil
- ➤ Juice of 1/2 lemon
- ➤ Salt and pepper to taste
- ➤ Cherry tomatoes for garnish

Instructions:

- ➤ In a food processor, combine basil leaves, pine nuts, garlic, Parmesan cheese (or nutritional yeast), olive oil, lemon juice, salt, and pepper. Pulse until smooth.
- ➤ Heat a large skillet over medium heat.
- ➤ Add zucchini noodles and cook for 2-3 minutes until just softened.
- ➤ Remove from heat and toss zucchini noodles with pesto sauce until evenly coated.

➤ Garnish with halved cherry tomatoes before serving.

Health Benefits:

➤ Zucchini is low in calories and carbohydrates, while basil provides vitamins and minerals.

➤ This dish is light, refreshing, and perfect for summer.

Preparation Time: 20 minutes

19: Butternut Squash Soup

Ingredients:

➤ 1 medium butternut squash, peeled, seeded, and diced

➤ 1 onion, diced

➤ 2 cloves garlic, minced

➤ 4 cups vegetable broth

➤ 1/2 teaspoon ground cinnamon

➤ 1/4 teaspoon ground nutmeg

➤ Salt and pepper to taste

➤ Coconut cream for garnish (optional)

Instructions:

➤ In a large pot, heat olive oil over medium heat.

➤ Add onion and garlic, sauté until softened.

- ➤ Add diced butternut squash, vegetable broth, cinnamon, and nutmeg.
- ➤ Bring to a boil, then reduce heat and simmer for 20-25 minutes until squash is tender.
- ➤ Use an immersion blender to puree the soup until smooth.
- ➤ Season with salt and pepper to taste.
- ➤ Serve hot, garnished with a drizzle of coconut cream if desired.

Health Benefits:

- ➤ Butternut squash is rich in vitamins A and C, while cinnamon and nutmeg add warmth and flavor.
- ➤ This soup is creamy, comforting, and perfect for chilly days.

Preparation Time: 40 minutes

20: Banana Oatmeal Pancakes

Ingredients:

- ➤ 1 ripe banana, mashed
- ➤ 1 cup rolled oats

- ➢ 1/2 cup unsweetened almond milk (or any plant-based milk)
- ➢ 1 tablespoon maple syrup
- ➢ 1 teaspoon vanilla extract
- ➢ 1/2 teaspoon ground cinnamon
- ➢ 1/2 teaspoon baking powder
- ➢ Pinch of salt
- ➢ Coconut oil or cooking spray for greasing the pan
- ➢ Fresh berries and maple syrup for serving

Instructions:

- ➢ In a blender or food processor, combine mashed banana, rolled oats, almond milk, maple syrup, vanilla extract, cinnamon, baking powder, and salt. Blend until smooth.
- ➢ Heat a non-stick skillet or griddle over medium heat and lightly grease with coconut oil or cooking spray.
- ➢ Pour pancake batter onto the skillet, using about 1/4 cup for each pancake.
- ➢ Cook until bubbles form on the surface of the pancakes, then flip and cook until golden brown on the other side.
- ➢ Repeat with the remaining batter.

> Serve pancakes hot with fresh berries and a drizzle of maple syrup.

Health Benefits:

> These pancakes are made with wholesome ingredients like bananas and oats, providing fiber, vitamins, and minerals.
> They're a nutritious and delicious breakfast option that's easy to make.

Preparation Time: 15 minutes

21: Mediterranean Quinoa Salad

Ingredients:

> 1 cup cooked quinoa
> 1 cup cherry tomatoes, halved
> 1 cucumber, diced
> 1/4 cup Kalamata olives, sliced
> 1/4 cup crumbled feta cheese (optional)
> 2 tablespoons chopped fresh parsley
> 2 tablespoons extra virgin olive oil
> 1 tablespoon lemon juice
> Salt and pepper to taste

Instructions:

> In a large bowl, combine cooked quinoa, cherry tomatoes, cucumber, Kalamata olives, and crumbled feta cheese.
> Drizzle with olive oil and lemon juice.
> Add chopped parsley and toss until well combined.
> Season with salt and pepper to taste.
> Serve chilled or at room temperature.

Health Benefits:

> This salad is packed with protein, fiber, vitamins, and minerals from quinoa, vegetables, and olives.
> It's light, refreshing, and perfect for summer.

Preparation Time: 20 minutes

22: Veggie Wrap

Ingredients:

> 1 large whole grain tortilla or wrap
> 2 tablespoons hummus
> 1/2 cup mixed salad greens
> 1/4 cup shredded carrots
> 1/4 cup sliced cucumber

> 1/4 cup sliced bell peppers

> 1/4 cup sliced avocado

> Salt and pepper to taste

Instructions:

> Lay the tortilla flat on a clean surface.

> Spread hummus evenly over the tortilla.

> Layer salad greens, shredded carrots, cucumber, bell peppers, and avocado on top of the hummus.

> Season with salt and pepper to taste.

> Roll up the tortilla tightly, tucking in the sides as you go.

> Slice the wrap in half diagonally.

> Serve immediately or wrap in foil for later.

Health Benefits:

> This veggie wrap is loaded with fiber, vitamins, and minerals from vegetables and whole grains.

> It's a convenient and portable meal option for on-the-go.

Preparation Time: 10 minutes

Ingredients:

- 1 head cauliflower, cut into florets
- 1/2 cup whole wheat flour (or chickpea flour for gluten-free option)
- 1/2 cup water
- 1 teaspoon garlic powder
- 1 teaspoon onion powder
- 1/2 teaspoon smoked paprika
- 1/4 teaspoon salt
- 1/4 teaspoon black pepper
- 1/2 cup buffalo sauce
- Ranch or blue cheese dressing for dipping (optional)

Instructions:

- Preheat oven to 450°F (230°C). Line a baking sheet with parchment paper.
- In a large bowl, whisk together whole wheat flour, water, garlic powder, onion powder, smoked paprika, salt, and black pepper to create a batter.
- Dip cauliflower florets into the batter, coating evenly, then place them on the prepared baking sheet.

- Bake for 20-25 minutes until cauliflower is tender and batter is crispy.
- Remove cauliflower from the oven and toss with buffalo sauce until evenly coated.
- Return cauliflower to the oven and bake for another 5-10 minutes until sauce is heated through.
- Serve hot with ranch or blue cheese dressing for dipping.

Health Benefits:

- Cauliflower is low in calories and high in fiber, vitamins, and minerals.
- This recipe provides a healthier alternative to traditional buffalo wings.

Preparation Time: 35 minutes

24: Vegan Lentil Tacos

Ingredients:

- 1 cup cooked lentils
- 1 tablespoon olive oil
- 1 onion, diced
- 2 cloves garlic, minced

- ➢ 1 bell pepper, diced
- ➢ 1 tablespoon chili powder
- ➢ 1 teaspoon ground cumin
- ➢ 1/2 teaspoon smoked paprika
- ➢ Salt and pepper to taste
- ➢ 8 small corn tortillas
- ➢ Toppings: diced avocado, salsa, shredded lettuce, lime wedges

Instructions:

- ➢ Heat olive oil in a skillet over medium heat.
- ➢ Add onion, garlic, and bell pepper. Sauté until softened.
- ➢ Stir in cooked lentils, chili powder, cumin, smoked paprika, salt, and pepper. Cook for another 5 minutes until heated through.
- ➢ Warm corn tortillas in the oven or on a skillet.
- ➢ Assemble tacos with lentil mixture and desired toppings.
- ➢ Serve with lime wedges.

Health Benefits:Lentils are rich in protein and fiber, while vegetables provide vitamins and minerals.

➢ Corn tortillas are gluten-free and high in fiber.

Preparation Time: 25 minutes

25: Spinach and Feta Stuffed Mushrooms

Ingredients:

➢ 12 large button mushrooms, stems removed and reserved
➢ 2 cups fresh spinach leaves, chopped
➢ 1/4 cup diced onion
➢ 2 cloves garlic, minced
➢ 1/4 cup crumbled feta cheese
➢ 1 tablespoon olive oil
➢ Salt and pepper to taste

Instructions:

➢ Preheat oven to 375°F (190°C). Line a baking sheet with parchment paper.
➢ Finely chop the reserved mushroom stems.
➢ Heat olive oil in a skillet over medium heat.
➢ Add chopped mushroom stems, onion, and garlic. Sauté until softened.
➢ Add chopped spinach and cook until wilted.

- ➢ Remove skillet from heat and stir in crumbled feta cheese. Season with salt and pepper to taste.
- ➢ Fill each mushroom cap with the spinach mixture and place them on the prepared baking sheet.
- ➢ Bake for 15-20 minutes until mushrooms are tender and filling is golden brown.
- ➢ Serve hot as an appetizer or side dish.

Health Benefits:

- ➢ Mushrooms are low in calories and rich in vitamins and minerals, while spinach provides iron and antioxidants.
- ➢ This dish is flavorful and nutrient-dense.

Preparation Time: 30 minutes

26: Tofu Scramble

Ingredients:

- ➢ 1 block firm tofu, drained and crumbled
- ➢ 1 tablespoon olive oil
- ➢ 1/2 onion, diced
- ➢ 1 bell pepper, diced
- ➢ 2 cloves garlic, minced

- ➢ 1 teaspoon ground turmeric
- ➢ 1/2 teaspoon ground cumin
- ➢ Salt and pepper to taste
- ➢ Fresh parsley for garnish (optional)

Instructions:

- ➢ Heat olive oil in a skillet over medium heat.
- ➢ Add onion, bell pepper, and garlic. Sauté until softened.
- ➢ Add crumbled tofu to the skillet. Cook for 5-7 minutes, stirring occasionally.
- ➢ Stir in ground turmeric, ground cumin, salt, and pepper. Cook for another 2-3 minutes until tofu is heated through and coated with spices.
- ➢ Garnish with fresh parsley if desired.
- ➢ Serve hot with toast or tortillas.

Health Benefits:

- ➢ Tofu is a source of plant-based protein, while vegetables provide vitamins and minerals.
- ➢ This tofu scramble is a satisfying and nutritious breakfast option.

Preparation Time: 15 minutes

27: Vegetable Frittata

Ingredients:

- 8 large eggs
- 1/4 cup milk (dairy or plant-based)
- 1 cup mixed vegetables (bell peppers, spinach, tomatoes)
- 1/2 cup shredded cheese (cheddar, mozzarella, or dairy-free cheese)
- 2 tablespoons olive oil
- Salt and pepper to taste
- Fresh herbs for garnish (optional)

Instructions:

- Preheat oven to 350°F (175°C).
- In a mixing bowl, whisk together eggs and milk. Season with salt and pepper.
- Heat olive oil in an oven-safe skillet over medium heat.
- Add mixed vegetables to the skillet and sauté until softened.
- Pour the egg mixture over the vegetables in the skillet. Sprinkle shredded cheese on top.

- Cook for 3-4 minutes until the edges begin to set.
- Transfer the skillet to the preheated oven and bake for 15-20 minutes until the frittata is cooked through and golden brown on top.
- Remove from the oven and let it cool slightly before slicing.
- Garnish with fresh herbs if desired.
- Serve warm or at room temperature.

Health Benefits:

- Eggs provide protein and essential nutrients, while vegetables offer vitamins and minerals.
- This vegetable frittata is versatile and can be enjoyed for breakfast, lunch, or dinner.

Preparation Time: 30 minutes

28: Roasted Vegetable Buddha Bowl

Ingredients:

- 1 cup cooked quinoa or brown rice
- 2 cups mixed vegetables (sweet potatoes, broccoli, cauliflower)
- 2 tablespoons olive oil

- ➢ 1 teaspoon garlic powder
- ➢ 1 teaspoon smoked paprika
- ➢ Salt and pepper to taste
- ➢ Tahini dressing for serving

Instructions:

- ➢ Preheat oven to 425°F (220°C). Line a baking sheet with parchment paper.
- ➢ Cut mixed vegetables into bite-sized pieces and place them on the prepared baking sheet.
- ➢ Drizzle olive oil over the vegetables and sprinkle with garlic powder, smoked paprika, salt, and pepper. Toss until evenly coated.
- ➢ Roast vegetables in the preheated oven for 20-25 minutes until tender and golden brown.
- ➢ Divide cooked quinoa or brown rice among serving bowls.
- ➢ Top with roasted vegetables.
- ➢ Drizzle with tahini dressing before serving.

Health Benefits:

This Buddha bowl is packed with fiber, vitamins, and minerals from quinoa, vegetables, and tahini dressing.

> It's a satisfying and nutritious meal option.

Preparation Time: 35 minutes

29: Caprese Salad

Ingredients:

- 2 large tomatoes, sliced
- 1 ball fresh mozzarella cheese, sliced
- Fresh basil leaves
- 2 tablespoons extra virgin olive oil
- 1 tablespoon balsamic glaze
- Salt and pepper to taste

Instructions:

- Arrange tomato slices and mozzarella slices alternately on a serving platter.
- Tuck fresh basil leaves between the tomato and mozzarella slices.
- Drizzle extra virgin olive oil and balsamic glaze over the salad.
- Season with salt and pepper to taste.
- Serve immediately as a refreshing appetizer or side dish.

Health Benefits:

> - Tomatoes are rich in vitamins and antioxidants, while fresh mozzarella provides protein and calcium.
> - This Caprese salad is light, flavorful, and perfect for summer.

Preparation Time: 10 minutes

30: Blueberry Chia Pudding

Ingredients:

> - 1/4 cup chia seeds
> - 1 cup unsweetened almond milk (or any plant-based milk)
> - 1 tablespoon maple syrup
> - 1/2 teaspoon vanilla extract
> - 1/2 cup fresh blueberries
> - Optional toppings: sliced almonds, shredded coconut

Instructions:

> - In a mixing bowl, whisk together chia seeds, almond milk, maple syrup, and vanilla extract.
> - Let the mixture sit for 5 minutes, then whisk again to break up any clumps.

- ➢ Cover the bowl and refrigerate for at least 2 hours or overnight until the chia pudding has thickened.
- ➢ Before serving, stir in fresh blueberries.
- ➢ Divide the chia pudding into serving bowls and top with optional toppings like sliced almonds or shredded coconut.

Health Benefits:

- ➢ Chia seeds are rich in fiber, omega-3 fatty acids, and antioxidants, while blueberries provide vitamins and minerals.
- ➢ This pudding is a nutritious and satisfying dessert or snack option.

Preparation Time: 5 minutes (plus chilling time)

31: Roasted Beet and Goat Cheese Salad

Ingredients:

- ➢ 2 medium beets, peeled and diced
- ➢ 2 tablespoons olive oil
- ➢ Salt and pepper to taste
- ➢ 4 cups mixed salad greens
- ➢ 1/4 cup crumbled goat cheese

- ➢ 2 tablespoons balsamic glaze
- ➢ Optional: toasted walnuts or pecans for garnish

Instructions:

- ➢ Preheat oven to 400°F (200°C). Line a baking sheet with parchment paper.
- ➢ Place diced beets on the prepared baking sheet. Drizzle with olive oil and season with salt and pepper. Toss until evenly coated.
- ➢ Roast beets in the preheated oven for 20-25 minutes until tender and caramelized.
- ➢ In a large bowl, toss mixed salad greens with roasted beets and crumbled goat cheese.
- ➢ Drizzle balsamic glaze over the salad and toss until well combined.
- ➢ Garnish with toasted walnuts or pecans if desired.
- ➢ Serve immediately as a vibrant and flavorful salad.

Health Benefits:

- ➢ Beets are high in fiber, vitamins, and antioxidants, while goat cheese provides protein and calcium.
- ➢ This salad is a delicious and nutritious option for lunch or dinner.

Preparation Time: 30 minutes

32: Veggie and Hummus Wrap

Ingredients:

- 1 large whole grain tortilla or wrap
- 2 tablespoons hummus
- 1/2 cup mixed salad greens
- 1/4 cup shredded carrots
- 1/4 cup sliced cucumber
- 1/4 cup sliced bell peppers
- 1/4 cup sliced avocado
- Salt and pepper to taste

Instructions:

- Lay the tortilla flat on a clean surface.
- Spread hummus evenly over the tortilla.
- Layer salad greens, shredded carrots, cucumber, bell peppers, and avocado on top of the hummus.
- Season with salt and pepper to taste.
- Roll up the tortilla tightly, tucking in the sides as you go.
- Slice the wrap in half diagonally.
- Serve immediately or wrap in foil for later.

Health Benefits:

> ➢ This veggie wrap is loaded with fiber, vitamins, and minerals from vegetables and whole grains.
> ➢ It's a convenient and portable meal option for on-the-go.

Preparation Time: 10 minutes

33: Coconut Curry Lentil Soup

Ingredients:

> ➢ 1 cup dried red lentils
> ➢ 1 tablespoon coconut oil
> ➢ 1 onion, diced
> ➢ 2 cloves garlic, minced
> ➢ 1 tablespoon grated fresh ginger
> ➢ 2 tablespoons curry powder
> ➢ 1 can (14 ounces) coconut milk
> ➢ 4 cups vegetable broth
> ➢ 2 cups chopped vegetables (carrots, sweet potatoes, spinach)
> ➢ Juice of 1 lime
> ➢ Salt and pepper to taste
> ➢ Fresh cilantro for garnish

Instructions:

- ➢ Rinse red lentils under cold water until the water runs clear. Drain and set aside.
- ➢ Heat coconut oil in a large pot over medium heat.
- ➢ Add diced onion, minced garlic, and grated ginger. Sauté until fragrant.
- ➢ Stir in curry powder and cook for 1 minute.
- ➢ Add coconut milk, vegetable broth, and red lentils to the pot. Bring to a boil.
- ➢ Reduce heat to low and simmer for 20-25 minutes until lentils are tender.
- ➢ Stir in chopped vegetables and continue to simmer for another 10 minutes until vegetables are cooked.
- ➢ Remove from heat and stir in lime juice. Season with salt and pepper to taste.
- ➢ Garnish with fresh cilantro before serving.

Health Benefits:

- ➢ Red lentils are rich in protein and fiber, while coconut milk provides healthy fats.
- ➢ This soup is creamy, flavorful, and nourishing.

Preparation Time: 45 minutes

34: Quinoa Black Bean Salad

Ingredients:

- 1 cup cooked quinoa
- 1 can black beans, drained and rinsed
- 1 cup corn kernels (fresh, frozen, or canned)
- 1 bell pepper, diced
- 1/4 cup diced red onion
- 1/4 cup chopped fresh cilantro
- Juice of 1 lime
- 2 tablespoons olive oil
- 1 teaspoon ground cumin
- Salt and pepper to taste
- Avocado slices for serving

Instructions:

- In a large bowl, combine cooked quinoa, black beans, corn kernels, diced bell pepper, red onion, and chopped cilantro.
- In a small bowl, whisk together lime juice, olive oil, ground cumin, salt, and pepper to make the dressing.

- ➢ Pour the dressing over the quinoa salad and toss until well combined.
- ➢ Serve chilled or at room temperature with avocado slices on top.

Health Benefits:

- ➢ Quinoa and black beans provide protein and fiber, while vegetables offer vitamins and minerals.
- ➢ This salad is refreshing, satisfying, and perfect for meal prep.

Preparation Time: 20 minutes

35: Sweet Potato and Black Bean Tacos

Ingredients:

- ➢ 2 large sweet potatoes, peeled and diced
- ➢ 1 tablespoon olive oil
- ➢ 1 teaspoon chili powder
- ➢ 1/2 teaspoon ground cumin
- ➢ 1/2 teaspoon smoked paprika
- ➢ Salt and pepper to taste
- ➢ 1 can black beans, drained and rinsed
- ➢ 8 small corn tortillas

➢ Toppings: diced avocado, salsa, shredded lettuce, lime wedges

Instructions:

➢ Preheat oven to 400°F (200°C). Line a baking sheet with parchment paper.

➢ In a large bowl, toss diced sweet potatoes with olive oil, chili powder, cumin, smoked paprika, salt, and pepper until evenly coated.

➢ Spread sweet potatoes in a single layer on the prepared baking sheet.

➢ Roast in the preheated oven for 20-25 minutes until tender and caramelized.

➢ In a small saucepan, heat black beans over medium heat until warmed through.

➢ Warm corn tortillas in the oven or on a skillet.

➢ Assemble tacos with roasted sweet potatoes, black beans, and desired toppings.

➢ Serve with lime wedges.

Health Benefits:

➢ Sweet potatoes are rich in vitamins and antioxidants, while black beans provide protein and fiber.

➢ These tacos are flavorful, satisfying, and perfect for a meatless meal.

Preparation Time: 30 minutes

36: Spinach and Mushroom Quesadillas

Ingredients:

- ➢ 4 large flour tortillas
- ➢ 2 cups fresh spinach leaves
- ➢ 1 cup sliced mushrooms
- ➢ 1/2 cup shredded cheese (cheddar, mozzarella, or dairy-free cheese)
- ➢ 2 tablespoons olive oil
- ➢ Salt and pepper to taste
- ➢ Salsa and Greek yogurt or sour cream for serving

Instructions:

- ➢ Heat olive oil in a large skillet over medium heat.
- ➢ Add sliced mushrooms and sauté until golden brown.
- ➢ Add fresh spinach leaves to the skillet and cook until wilted. Season with salt and pepper to taste.
- ➢ Remove mushrooms and spinach from the skillet and set aside.

- ➤ Place a flour tortilla in the skillet. Sprinkle shredded cheese evenly over the tortilla.
- ➤ Layer cooked mushrooms and spinach on one half of the tortilla.
- ➤ Fold the other half of the tortilla over the filling to create a half-moon shape.
- ➤ Cook quesadilla for 2-3 minutes on each side until golden brown and crispy.
- ➤ Repeat with the remaining tortillas and filling.
- ➤ Slice quesadillas into wedges and serve hot with salsa and Greek yogurt or sour cream.

Health Benefits:

- ➤ Spinach is rich in iron and vitamins, while mushrooms provide antioxidants.
- ➤ These quesadillas are a quick and easy meal option for lunch or dinner.

Preparation Time: 20 minutes

37: Black Bean and Corn Salad

Ingredients:

- ➤ 1 can black beans, drained and rinsed

- 1 cup corn kernels (fresh, frozen, or canned)
- 1/2 cup diced bell pepper
- 1/4 cup diced red onion
- 2 tablespoons chopped fresh cilantro
- Juice of 1 lime
- 1 tablespoon olive oil
- 1/2 teaspoon ground cumin
- Salt and pepper to taste
- Avocado slices for serving

Instructions:

- In a large bowl, combine black beans, corn kernels, diced bell pepper, red onion, and chopped cilantro.
- In a small bowl, whisk together lime juice, olive oil, ground cumin, salt, and pepper to make the dressing.
- Pour the dressing over the black bean salad and toss until well combined.
- Serve chilled or at room temperature with avocado slices on top.

Health Benefits:

- Black beans are rich in protein and fiber, while vegetables provide vitamins and minerals.

- This salad is light, refreshing, and perfect for picnics or potlucks.

Preparation Time: 15 minutes

38: Broccoli and Cheddar Soup

Ingredients:

- 4 cups broccoli florets
- 1 onion, diced
- 2 cloves garlic, minced
- 4 cups vegetable broth
- 1 cup shredded cheddar cheese (or dairy-free cheese)
- 1/2 cup heavy cream (or coconut cream for vegan option)
- Salt and pepper to taste
- Croutons for garnish (optional)

Instructions:

- In a large pot, heat olive oil over medium heat.
- Add diced onion and minced garlic. Sauté until softened.
- Add broccoli florets and vegetable broth to the pot. Bring to a boil.

➤ Reduce heat to low and simmer for 15-20 minutes until broccoli is tender.

➤ Use an immersion blender to puree the soup until smooth.

➤ Stir in shredded cheddar cheese and heavy cream until cheese is melted.

➤ Season with salt and pepper to taste.

➤ Serve hot with croutons for garnish if desired.

Health Benefits:

➤ Broccoli is rich in vitamins and antioxidants, while cheddar cheese provides calcium and protein.

➤ This soup is creamy, comforting, and perfect for chilly days.

Preparation Time: 30 minutes

39: Stuffed Bell Peppers

Ingredients:

➤ 4 large bell peppers, halved and seeds removed

➤ 1 cup cooked quinoa

➤ 1 can black beans, drained and rinsed

➤ 1 cup corn kernels (fresh, frozen, or canned)

- ➤ 1 cup diced tomatoes
- ➤ 1/2 cup diced red onion
- ➤ 1 teaspoon chili powder
- ➤ 1/2 teaspoon cumin
- ➤ Salt and pepper to taste
- ➤ Shredded cheese or nutritional yeast for topping

Instructions:

- ➤ Preheat oven to 375°F (190°C).
- ➤ In a large mixing bowl, combine cooked quinoa, black beans, corn, diced tomatoes, red onion, chili powder, cumin, salt, and pepper.
- ➤ Place bell pepper halves in a baking dish, cut side up.
- ➤ Spoon quinoa mixture into each pepper half until filled.
- ➤ Cover the baking dish with aluminum foil and bake for 30-35 minutes until peppers are tender.
- ➤ Remove foil, sprinkle shredded cheese or nutritional yeast on top of each stuffed pepper, and return to the oven for another 5 minutes until cheese is melted.
- ➤ Serve hot.

Health Benefits:

> ➤ Bell peppers are rich in vitamins and antioxidants, while quinoa and black beans provide protein and fiber.
> ➤ This dish is colorful, flavorful, and nutrient-packed.

Preparation Time: 45 minutes

40: Veggie Stir-Fry

Ingredients:

> ➤ 2 cups mixed vegetables (bell peppers, broccoli, carrots, snap peas)
> ➤ 1 tablespoon sesame oil
> ➤ 2 cloves garlic, minced
> ➤ 1 tablespoon grated fresh ginger
> ➤ 1/4 cup soy sauce (or tamari for gluten-free option)
> ➤ 1 tablespoon rice vinegar
> ➤ 1 tablespoon maple syrup (or honey)
> ➤ 2 teaspoons cornstarch
> ➤ Cooked brown rice or quinoa for serving

Instructions: Heat sesame oil in a large skillet or wok over medium-high heat.

- ➢ Add minced garlic and grated ginger to the skillet. Sauté until fragrant.
- ➢ Add mixed vegetables to the skillet and stir-fry until tender-crisp.
- ➢ In a small bowl, whisk together soy sauce, rice vinegar, maple syrup, and cornstarch to make the sauce.
- ➢ Pour the sauce over the vegetables in the skillet. Stir until evenly coated.
- ➢ Cook for another 2-3 minutes until the sauce has thickened.
- ➢ Serve hot over cooked brown rice or quinoa.

Health Benefits:

- ➢ Mixed vegetables provide vitamins, minerals, and fiber, while sesame oil adds flavor and healthy fats.
- ➢ This stir-fry is quick, easy, and customizable with your favorite veggies.

Preparation Time: 20 minutes

CONCLUSION

Embarking on a journey towards a vegetarian diet tailored to manage Sjogren's syndrome can be both rewarding and empowering.

Through this cookbook for beginners, we've delved into a world of delicious, nutritious, and easy-to-prepare recipes that not only cater to the specific dietary needs of seniors dealing with Sjogren's syndrome but also promote overall health and well-being.

From hearty breakfasts to satisfying lunches, flavorful dinners, and delightful snacks, each recipe has been thoughtfully crafted to provide a balance of essential nutrients while tantalizing the taste buds with vibrant flavors and textures.

By incorporating a variety of wholesome ingredients such as fruits, vegetables, legumes, whole grains, and plant-based proteins, these recipes aim to nourish the body and support optimal health. Moreover, this cookbook serves as a guide, offering valuable insights, tips, and guidelines for navigating the principles of vegetarianism in managing Sjogren's syndrome.

Whether you're seeking relief from symptoms, aiming to improve your overall health, or simply looking to explore the benefits of plant-based eating, these recipes provide a solid foundation for embarking on your culinary journey.

As you embark on this path towards wellness, remember that every meal is an opportunity to nourish your body, indulge your senses, and embrace the joy of cooking.

May this cookbook inspire you to discover new flavors, expand your culinary horizons, and embark on a journey towards vibrant health and vitality.

Cheers to good health, happy cooking, and delicious meals shared with loved ones!